INVISIBLE STRENGTH: A JOURNEY OF RESILIENCE WITH HIV

By

Richard J. Martin, CTSS

Copyright Page

Dedication

To every soul navigating the journey of an HIV diagnosis—this book is dedicated to you, to your strength, and to the courage it takes to rewrite the story and redefine what it means to live with HIV.

Since March 23, 2007, HIV has lived with me. It has not always been that way; at first, it felt like I was the one living under its shadow, confined by fear and the weight of stigma. I was bullied by it, as much by the world around me as by the uncertainty within. There were moments when I felt like a victim, trapped by my own body and society's relentless judgment. I know the isolation, the whispered assumptions, the constant vigilance of wondering if others "see" it even when it is invisible.

However, somewhere along this path, I discovered something powerful: the strength to regain control and reclaim my life and identity. Over time, I turned the language around. I decided that, no matter the diagnosis, I would be the one in control. I would not live in the shadow of HIV—it would live with me. I would not be defined by this virus nor let it dictate the boundaries of my life, dreams, or worth.

To anyone who has ever faced this journey and wondered how to move forward, I hope this story speaks to you. To those who have been crushed by stigma, who have felt invisible under the weight of judgment, may you find the power to stand tall, to live boldly, and to know that this journey is yours to command. I hope you know you can take ownership, shifting from "living with" to letting it simply "live with you." You have the power to rule it, to stand in your truth, and to let your story be one of survival, not submission.

This book is dedicated to everyone who has refused to be reduced by a diagnosis, those on their way to reclaiming their own stories, and those still searching for strength within. Know that you are resilient, courageous, and never alone.

You are SEEN!

You are WORTHY!

You are LOVED!

You are a CHAMPION!

You are VICTORIOUS!

GO AND RECLAIM YOUR LIFE.

Love and light

Richard J. Martin

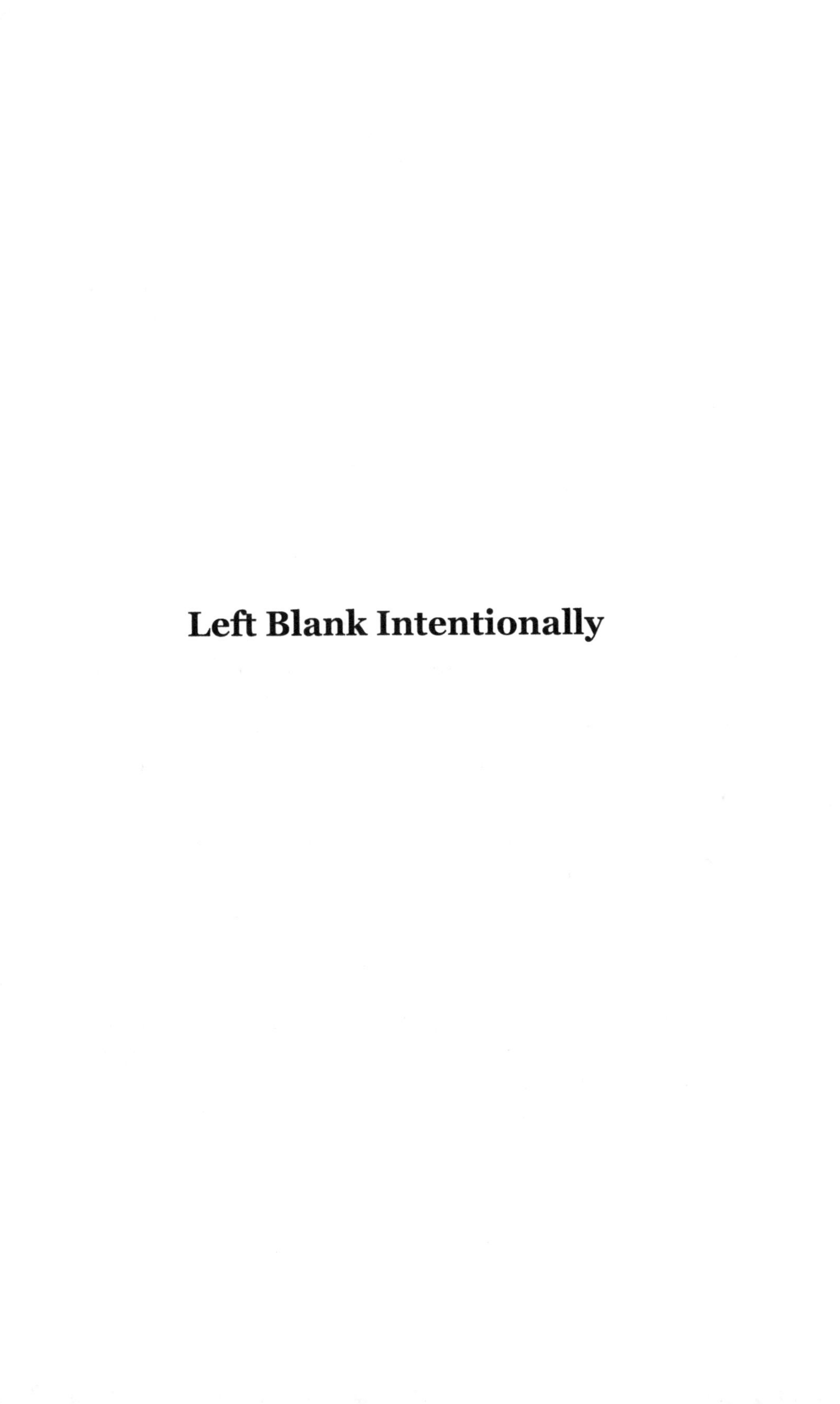

Left Blank Intentionally

Opening Prayer

Dear Creator of Life, Source of all Strength,

We come before you in humility and gratitude, seeking your presence and peace. We ask for the courage to face each day with resilience and the wisdom to see beyond the challenges we bear. Grant us the strength to remember that we are not defined by any single moment, diagnosis, or circumstance but by our enduring spirit.

May we find the grace to release shame and respectfully embrace our truth. Help us to walk in the light of acceptance, to let go of fear, and to see ourselves as you see us—whole, beloved, and worthy of all good things. In times of doubt, be our steadfast guide, reminding us of our strength, which endures beyond pain, stigma, and fear.

We pray for all those whose lives are touched by HIV, seen and unseen. Surround them with love, understanding, and the support of genuinely caring people. May they find peace knowing they are not alone and feel empowered to live boldly and authentically.

Guide us as we seek purpose in our journey and turn our struggles into stories of hope, advocacy, and love. May our experiences be a light to others, a testament that there is a way forward, even in the darkest times.

Let us find meaning in our resilience, courage in our vulnerability, and hope in the possibility of a life filled with joy, purpose, and connection. Walk with us, uplift us, and remind us that we are always in your loving embrace.

Amen. Amen. Amen.

Table of Contents

Introduction

Every life has moments that divide time into distinct "before" and "after." For Adrian, a compassionate, hard-working man with a steady life and modest dreams, that moment arrived with a doctor's simple but life-altering words: "You have HIV." With those words, everything he once understood about himself, his future, and his place in the world shifted. From that moment forward, HIV would live with him—a presence that might shape his life but one that he would refuse to let define him.

This story, inspired by real-world experiences, mirrors the journey that so many have taken since the early days of the HIV epidemic. Adrian's path is filled with intense emotions, from isolation and fear to resilience and rediscovering purpose. Each stage of his journey brings to light the hidden struggles that people diagnosed with HIV often bear in silence. Yet, it is equally a story of hope, of a man who learns that he is far more than a diagnosis and that resilience can emerge from even the darkest places.

Invisible Strength is more than a narrative about illness; it is a story of resilience, acceptance, and transformation. In many ways, Adrian's journey reflects the universal human need to belong, to love, and to live authentically despite the labels society imposes. This book walks us through the unique challenges Adrian faces as he learns to cope with the realities of having HIV live with him, confronts the stigma surrounding his condition, and ultimately transforms his pain into a source of strength—not only for himself but for others who face similar struggles.

For Adrian, the diagnosis initially brings devastation, the weight of shame, and the instinct to hide from a world that he fears will judge him. His relationships shift, some fading while others grow unexpectedly stronger. He faces the daily burden of decisions—who to tell, how much to reveal, and how to navigate the deeply personal challenge of finding acceptance within himself before seeking it from others.

Adrian's story is not a simple, linear progression from despair to hope. It is messy, layered, and, at times, painfully isolating. But it is within the complexity of this journey that he begins to reclaim his life. He moves from merely surviving to embracing his identity with pride, letting go of shame, and advocating for others. He learns that vulnerability is not a weakness but a pathway to connection. He comes to understand that while HIV lives with him, it does not have to rule or define his life.

Throughout the book, we follow Adrian as he stumbles, learns, and grows. His journey is told in ten chapters, each a window into his evolution from despair to resilience. In each chapter, Adrian faces new challenges, from confronting his fears and finding support to redefining his relationships and stepping into his role as an advocate. This book seeks to illuminate the emotional and mental dimensions of having HIV live with you—a story that too often goes untold, clouded by society's lingering stigmas and misconceptions.

For those reading who may walk a similar path, Adrian's story is a reminder that you are not alone. His struggles and triumphs echo the quiet courage within so many who refuse to be limited by HIV as it lives with them. For those unfamiliar with the experience, this story offers a compassionate glimpse into a life often misunderstood, an opportunity to see beyond the diagnosis to the person who lives with it.

Invisible Strength is an invitation to journey alongside Adrian, to feel his doubts, joys, despair, and victories. It is a testament to the power of resilience, the importance of understanding and empathy, and the human spirit's capacity to rise despite life's most daunting challenges. Adrian's story is for all of us—an acknowledgment that life, in its most difficult moments, holds the potential for profound transformation, growth, and unbreakable courage.

As you turn these pages, may you find the courage to face your challenges, the strength to support those around you, and the empathy to see beyond the surface of any diagnosis.

The Diagnosis

The Shock

Adrian had always considered himself healthy, with goals and a decent sense of direction. Sure, he'd had the occasional flu or a twisted ankle, but nothing had ever felt insurmountable, nothing that had shaken his sense of self. He was used to moving through life confidently, balancing work, friendships, and quiet ambitions until that day in the doctor's office; one conversation changed everything.

The doctor's voice sounded strangely distant, almost as if he were speaking through a tunnel. Adrian sat there, hands gripped tightly around the arms of his chair, trying to make sense of the words that hovered between them. "You have HIV." Three words that seemed to slice through him, leaving behind a numbness he'd never known. He had gone in expecting routine results, maybe a tiny admonishment about his caffeine intake, but nothing that would upend his entire understanding of himself.

At first, he felt disbelief, a solid wall of refusal that went up immediately. *He thought this couldn't be right,* almost as if he could undo the diagnosis by sheer will. This wasn't something that happened to him. HIV was something distant, something you read about in headlines or heard about from friends or friends. It wasn't supposed to be accurate, not like this. The disbelief gave way to a torrent of emotions, all colliding inside him with the force of a tidal wave—fear, shame, confusion, even anger. He wanted to reach for someone, but who could he call with news like this? And how could he possibly make them understand?

He barely remembered leaving the doctor's office, his legs moving him out of the building and onto the street by instinct alone. The city seemed to move around him, oblivious to the bombshell that had just dropped into his world. He wandered, unable to return to his apartment and face the normalcy of his belongings, the untouched dishes, and the books still marked by dog-eared pages from days before he'd ever considered this possibility.

That night, he lay in bed staring at the ceiling, the weight of his thoughts pressing down on him like a physical burden. He kept repeating the words in his mind, hoping they'd somehow lose their impact or fade into some distant nightmare he could shake off. *HIV lives with me.* The words hung there, immovable, a new reality he didn't yet know how to live with.

Doctor's Office Reality

The next few days passed in a blur of disconnected tasks. He went through the motions, yet his mind remained frozen at that moment in the doctor's office. Adrian knew he had to go back to face whatever this diagnosis meant and understand what it required of him. With equal parts dread and determination, he scheduled a follow-up appointment to learn more.

When he entered the doctor's office again, it felt as though he were stepping into the scene of an accident, reliving the impact of news he still couldn't fully grasp. His doctor explained the medical realities of HIV in calm, clinical terms. Adrian listened, nodding at intervals, his mind a swirl of technical words and figures. CD4 counts, viral load, antiretrovirals—a language he hadn't prepared to understand, a maze of information that felt impersonal and overwhelming.

He had questions, endless questions. Would this change how people saw him? Could he still live a "normal" life, or had that possibility vanished? He couldn't help but wonder if his doctor, in all his reassurance, truly understood the personal weight of this diagnosis. Each answer brought a flood of new fears, and Adrian left with more questions than when he had arrived. This was more than just a medical condition; it was a reality that demanded he face every assumption he'd ever had about himself and the life he'd imagined.

The Shame and the Stigma

As Adrian attempted to process his new reality, a different kind of weight began to settle in—one he hadn't anticipated. The social stigma around HIV began to color his perception of himself. He started to wonder how others would react if the world would see him differently and if friends or colleagues might withdraw if they knew. The whispers of judgment seemed to echo from the walls around him, though he hadn't told a soul.

He noticed his behavior shifting, the instinct to withdraw becoming almost automatic. He'd begun pulling away subtly, avoiding friends' messages, declining invitations to gatherings he'd typically enjoy. He was haunted by the thought that people might see him as damaged or contaminated, no longer the Adrian they knew. Society had so many unspoken rules and so many judgments. He could feel them pressing against him, reminding him that in their eyes, this diagnosis meant something more than just a virus—it meant shame.

Adrian grappled with this silently, feeling the crushing pressure of a world that often failed to understand and that too easily defined people by their conditions. The shame felt isolating, a private battle that left him afraid to look people in the eye, fearing they would somehow see his hidden truth.

Isolation Begins

Adrian's instinct to withdraw began to take over. At work, he kept conversations to a minimum, smiling politely but never lingering long enough for anyone to ask how he was doing. He isolated himself, retreating from even the closest of friends. He wanted to reach out, to talk about what he was going through, but how could he? The words felt foreign and heavy, a truth that might be too much for anyone to handle.

He began to feel like a stranger in his own life, watching from a distance as the world carried on without him. The walls of his apartment felt closer each night, his thoughts amplifying the feeling of being trapped. He was living with a secret he wasn't sure he could ever share. As he closed himself off, the isolation began to feed on itself, leaving him with a profound sense of loneliness.

Searching for Support

In time, Adrian realized that he couldn't carry this burden alone. He needed someone, anyone, who could understand. He started searching online, reading about support groups and forums for people with HIV. He found that there were others like him, people who had been living with HIV for years, some even thriving. Slowly, he began to understand that he wasn't as alone as he felt.

Attending his first support group meeting was both terrifying and relieving. He was surrounded by people who understood, had felt the same fear and shame, and had found a way to keep living. In their stories, he saw reflections of his journey, fragments of his fear and hopes. These people gave him something he hadn't felt in a long time: a glimmer of understanding and connection, the start of a path forward.

As Chapter 1 draws close, Adrian has just begun his journey. The shock of his diagnosis has shattered his world, but in his search for support, he has found the first threads of resilience. This new reality may be complex and painful, but he has discovered that others understand and will walk with him. Moreover, for the first time, he begins to believe that maybe, just maybe, he can reclaim his life from the grip of this diagnosis and learn to let HIV live with him instead of allowing it to rule him.

Living in the Shadows

Daily Fears

The days following Adrian's diagnosis were marked by an undercurrent of fear, a steady beat of anxiety that seemed to follow him everywhere. As he tried to settle back into his routine, he found that his mind rarely gave him a moment's rest. The world around him had not changed, but he felt everything about him had—his health, future, and sense of safety. With each passing day, he was consumed by a series of "what-ifs" that played on an endless loop, each one louder and more terrifying than the last.

He began to worry incessantly about his health, questioning every small change in his body, every moment of fatigue or slight ache. A simple headache became a cause for panic; a fleeting sore throat would send him spiraling. He no longer saw these as ordinary discomforts but potential signs of something catastrophic. He wondered if his body would betray him if HIV would suddenly decide to show itself in ways he could not control or predict. The paranoia grew, expanding from his physical health to his mental state. His mind seemed to turn against him, amplifying every fear and planting seeds of dread in places that used to bring him peace.

Once filled with quiet aspirations and personal goals, Adrian's future seemed blurry and uncertain. He had always taken life one step at a time, but now, each step felt weighed down by the unseen, the unknown. He questioned if he would ever find love if he could ever have a family, or if he was now consigned to a life of secrecy and solitude. It felt as though his diagnosis had stolen more than just his health—it had stolen his sense of possibility, leaving him stranded in a future that felt increasingly dark and limited.

The constant vigilance, the hyper-awareness of his own body, began to take a toll on him. His mind was a battlefield where hope and dread clashed constantly. He could no longer remember what it felt like to be carefree or spontaneous; every action and every thought was tinged with the presence of HIV, a silent but ever-looming presence in his life. The fear wrapped around him like a shadow, making it hard to breathe and to imagine a way forward that was not filled with anxiety.

Facing the Mirror

One morning, Adrian stood before his bathroom mirror, studying his reflection. His physical appearance had not changed; he looked the same as always. His hair was still dark and thick, his skin still clear. Outwardly, there was nothing different, no visible mark or sign that HIV was living with him. However, as he gazed at himself, he could not shake the feeling that something fundamental had shifted. It was as if his reflection were a stranger, someone wearing his face but burdened by a truth that could not be seen.

At that moment, Adrian felt deeply uncomfortable with his own body, a kind of betrayal he had not expected. He wondered if other people could sense it if there were some invisible marker that would give him away. Paranoia crept in as he walked through the world, feeling as though others might somehow "see" his diagnosis, even if, logically, he knew they could not. This sense of being on display, of being exposed, haunted him. He felt that his secret clung to him like a second skin, something he could never shed, no matter how much he wished to.

The mirror became both a comfort and a curse. It reminded him that he was still Adrian, still the same person. However, it also revealed his vulnerability and struggle to reconcile the person he had been with the person he was now. He looked into his eyes, searching for strength, for signs that he could still be whole. However, each time he did, he turned away, unable to bear the weight of his reflection. His self-image was fractured, and he feared that no one would ever see him the way he once was, that the presence of HIV would forever overshadow him.

Secrets and Lies

As Adrian's fears mounted, he slipped into a pattern of secrecy. Every interaction felt like a test, a careful dance around the truth that had taken over his life. He began to compartmentalize, separating parts of himself that he would allow others to see and those he would hide away. He avoided conversations that might lead to questions, topics that might inch too close to the truth. It was easier to deflect, change the subject, and mask his pain behind small talk and half-hearted smiles.

The lies were initially subtle—an excuse here, a vague answer there. However, he found himself actively hiding parts of his life over time. He felt the need to protect himself, to shield his friends and family from the reality that HIV now lived with him. He feared that if they knew, it would change everything—their perception of him would shift, and pity or judgment might taint how they loved and cared for him.

These secrets began to weigh on him, a quiet burden that made him feel even more isolated. He thought he was living two lives—one where he was still Adrian, still the friend and coworker they all knew, and another where he was someone new, someone they could not possibly understand. The secrecy became a wall, a barrier he could not breach, leaving him feeling lonelier than ever.

Rejection

In a moment of vulnerability, Adrian decided to confide in one of his closest friends, hoping that by sharing his truth, he might lighten the weight of his burden. He believed that if anyone could understand, it would be her; they had been through so much together, and he trusted her deeply. With trembling hands and a nervous heart, he told her the truth, revealing the presence of HIV in his life, hoping she might offer comfort, acceptance, or at least understanding.

However, her reaction was not what he had hoped for. Instead of empathy, he was met with discomfort, a strained silence that seemed to hang in the air. She pulled back, her face contorting with confusion, maybe even fear. She said she needed time and did not know how to process this. Her response stung, cutting into him in ways he had not expected. He felt he had been cast out and rejected by someone he thought would always be there.

The pain of her reaction left Adrian questioning his decision to be open, and it deepened his feelings of isolation. He withdrew further, convinced that his secret was too much for anyone to bear, that HIV had turned him into someone people could not accept. This rejection solidified his belief that he would have to face this alone, that his truth was a burden he could not share. The loneliness became more profound, a silent wound he carried with him, hidden beneath layers of forced smiles and guarded conversations.

A Glimmer of Hope

Amid this loneliness, Adrian met someone new whose warmth and kindness seemed genuine, unburdened by assumptions or fears. Their friendship began innocently, over shared laughter and casual conversations, but it became more meaningful. This person saw and spoke to him with respect and openness that he had not experienced in a long time. There was a lightness to their connection, a reminder that he could still be seen and valued for who he was.

As they spent more time together, Adrian began to feel a spark of hope. This friend did not know his diagnosis, but they saw him without judgment, without the shadow of HIV coloring their perception. Adrian realized that maybe, just maybe, there were people in the world who could look beyond a diagnosis, people who would accept him fully, with compassion and understanding. This new friendship began a small but powerful shift within him—a belief that he did not have to be alone and could still find connection, even if it meant taking the risk to be seen.

Chapter 2 closes with Adrian beginning to find a way forward. Though he still feels the weight of his fears, shame, and secrecy, he has found a glimmer of hope, a reminder that he is not beyond connection or love. This friendship is the first crack in the wall he has built around himself, a small light in the darkness that shows him a path forward. HIV may live with him, but he is beginning to see that it does not have to define every part of who he is.

The Weight of the World

Mental Health Battles

Adrian's days were marked by an unrelenting heaviness, a weight that seemed to settle deeper with every passing moment. Once a place of simple thoughts and occasional worries, his mind had become a storm of anxieties that left him feeling drained before getting out of bed. As he opened his eyes to the familiar sight of his room, a fresh wave of dread washed over him every morning. It was not just fear of his health or his future—it was an all-consuming ache, an invisible weight he could not lift or escape.

Anxiety and depression began to creep in, their effects settling into his mind and body like uninvited guests. Adrian found it challenging to concentrate at work, his thoughts clouded by worries he could not shake. Ordinary tasks became monumental, each one requiring an effort he barely possessed. Even simple acts—answering a phone call, making himself a meal, or responding to a text—felt overwhelming. His mind often drifted into dark spaces, places where hope felt like a distant, fading memory.

Sleep became both a refuge and an enemy. At night, he would lie awake, thoughts racing, replaying every fear and possible scenario of his future. When he finally drifted off, it was into a restless sleep filled with dreams that mirrored his real-life anxieties, leaving him exhausted each morning. The once-vibrant world around him now appeared muted and distant, his mind too preoccupied with a battle he could not explain or share.

Adrian began to recognize that his struggle was not just with HIV—it was with himself, with a mind that now seemed to betray him at every turn. He felt trapped in his thoughts, a prisoner to fears that grew stronger daily. This internal struggle became as exhausting as any physical battle, wearing him down in ways that made him feel helpless and hopeless. He had always thought of himself as resilient, but the depth of his mental and emotional anguish left him questioning that belief. How could he be resilient when he could not even find the strength to get through a single day without feeling overwhelmed?

A Search for Purpose

In the depths of his despair, Adrian realized he needed something to hold onto that could pull him out of the darkness that had taken over his life. He knew he could not continue like this, lost in a void of fears and self-doubt. He needed a reason to keep moving forward, a purpose that went beyond mere survival. Though unsure of where to start, he felt a flicker of hope in the idea that he could find meaning in his life once more.

He began to search for anything that could give him a sense of direction. In the past, he had been passionate about volunteering and spending weekends at local shelters and food banks. These activities had once filled him with a quiet satisfaction, a sense of giving back that grounded him. Now, he wondered if returning to such activities could help him reclaim a part of himself that had been lost.

The search for purpose was not easy. At times, Adrian felt foolish for thinking that volunteering or a new project could counterbalance the profound pain he carried. However, the simple act of searching, of imagining something beyond his current struggles, began to open a small space within him, a place where hope could retake root. He realized that purpose did not have to be grand or world-changing; it just had to be meaningful to him. Even in the most minor acts, he began to see the healing potential, a chance to rebuild his identity on his terms.

Faith and Spirituality

Adrian had always considered himself a person of faith, though not devout. Growing up, he had attended church with his family, absorbing the values and lessons that had shaped his understanding of the world. However, his faith had been quiet, a background presence rather than a guiding force. In the face of his struggles, he searched for comfort and answers in a realm he had not visited in years.

He intentionally explored his spirituality, seeking solace in prayer, meditation, and reading. At first, he hoped that faith might provide a sense of peace, a way to ground himself amidst the chaos of his mind. However, as he delved deeper, he found that his journey was filled with questions rather than answers. He questioned why he had to endure this struggle, why he felt so alone, and why he had to live with a diagnosis that felt like a life sentence.

Adrian wrestled with the tension between faith and reality. There were days when he felt a comforting presence, a sense that he was not alone in his suffering. On other days, he only felt silence, an emptiness that left him questioning everything he believed. His relationship with faith became both a comfort and a challenge, a source of guidance that demanded he confront his most profound doubts and fears.

In this spiritual exploration, Adrian found that his faith did not have to be perfect; it did not have to provide all the answers. It was enough that it was there, a small light in the darkness, a reminder that he was part of something greater than himself. His spirituality offered him moments of calm, and though fleeting, these moments became precious— glimpses of peace amidst the storm.

First Steps to Healing

Recognizing the toll his mental battles were taking, Adrian took a tentative step toward professional help. He scheduled his first appointment with a therapist, uncertain but hopeful that this might be a way forward. He had always prided himself on independence and handling his struggles alone. Admitting that he needed help felt vulnerable, almost like conceding defeat. However, he knew he could not continue carrying this weight alone.

In therapy, Adrian began to explore the roots of his pain, unraveling the complex emotions surrounding his diagnosis and the isolation it had brought. He spoke about the shame, the loneliness, the fear of rejection, and the constant, gnawing worry about his future. His therapist offered him a safe space to voice these fears, to lay bare the thoughts that had haunted him in silence. It was a relief to speak openly, to share his burdens with someone who would not judge or turn away.

He also began attending a support group, a small circle of individuals who understood his struggles without explanation. Each meeting brought new perspectives, stories of resilience, and an unspoken bond that connected them through their shared experiences. These people, each with their battles, showed Adrian that healing was possible and that he was not the only one carrying this weight.

The healing journey was slow, marked by small steps rather than grand transformations. However, Adrian felt less alone and hopeful with each therapy session and support group meeting. He began to see that healing was not about erasing pain but about finding a way to live alongside it, to carry it with grace rather than despair.

The Power of Empathy

As Adrian became more open to the stories of others, he found himself deeply moved by their experiences. Each person in his support group carried their burdens and had walked a path mirrored his. He listened to their stories of rejection, acceptance, struggle, and triumph, feeling an empathy he had not known. These people were not just strangers but reflections of his journey, each holding a piece of the truth he sought.

Through these connections, Adrian realized he was not alone in his pain. Others had faced similar fears, felt the same shame, and struggled with the same doubts. Their resilience inspired him, and their openness reminded him of the strength in vulnerability. By hearing their stories, he found himself less consumed by his struggles, his heart opening to a broader understanding of what it meant to live with HIV.

Empathy became a lifeline for Adrian to connect with others and himself. He saw that his personal pain was part of a larger story—a story of human resilience, of people finding ways to thrive despite their struggles. In this shared journey, Adrian found hope. He began to see his own life through a new lens, one that was no longer defined solely by his diagnosis but by his capacity to connect, understand, and heal.

As Chapter 3 comes to an end, Adrian has begun the complex but hopeful process of healing. His mental health struggles remain, but through therapy, faith, and empathy, he has found small but significant steps forward. He no longer carries the world's weight alone; he has discovered a community, a purpose, and a growing sense of peace. This chapter marks the beginning of a new phase in his journey—one of self-discovery, acceptance, and the quiet resilience that emerges when we allow others to walk alongside us in our pain.

Facing the Stigma Head-On

Confrontation

Adrian had become accustomed to managing his diagnosis quietly, his interactions and movements shaped by discretion and caution. He had spent months guarding his secret, controlling what he could to avoid judgment or pity. However, despite his best efforts, there were things he could not control—chief among them the prejudice in the world around him.

One afternoon, that prejudice erupted in a way that forced him to confront it head-on. He was at a neighborhood café, a place he frequented when he needed a quiet moment to think. He overheard a conversation at a nearby table as he ordered his coffee. A group was discussing HIV, throwing around outdated stereotypes, and casually making jokes that cut into him like a sharp edge. Their voices were filled with ignorance, and their words carried a disdain that shook him to his core. He felt his body tense, his hands trembling slightly as he clutched his coffee cup, unsure if he should speak up or walk away.

At that moment, something inside him snapped. He could no longer sit by and allow ignorance to dictate the narrative around HIV. For months, he had hidden, carried shame, and distanced himself to avoid this kind of confrontation. However, as he stood there, hearing his own life reduced to caricature and misinformation, he felt a surge of resolve, a need to speak not only for himself but for others who had been silenced by stigma.

Without fully thinking it through, Adrian approached their table. His voice was steady, though his heart raced with nerves. He challenged their misconceptions calmly and clearly, sharing that HIV did not make people "dirty" or "dangerous," as they had suggested. He explained that modern medicine allowed people with HIV to live whole lives and that ignorance was the actual danger—not the virus itself. As he spoke, he saw the surprise in their eyes, the realization that they had not expected to be called out, especially by someone with firsthand knowledge.

The exchange was brief, but it was enough. He walked away from the café, feeling an unexpected sense of pride. By confronting that small group, he had taken a stand against a prejudice he had internalized for so long. He realized that by letting stigma rule his life, he had, in a way, accepted it as valid. However, now, he saw that he had the power to push back, to challenge the narratives that had haunted him. It was a pivotal moment, one that ignited within him a fierce determination to fight the stigma surrounding HIV, both for himself and for others.

Educating Others

Inspired by his confrontation at the café, Adrian began thinking of ways to make a difference beyond single encounters. He wanted to help people understand the realities of HIV, to break down the walls of ignorance that separated people like him from the compassion they deserved. However, the idea of sharing his story openly felt daunting. There was a part of him that still feared judgment, that still wrestled with the desire to keep his diagnosis private.

After much thought, he decided to start an anonymous blog. Writing had always been a way for him to process his thoughts, and he realized that sharing his story, even anonymously, could allow him to reach others without exposing himself entirely. He crafted his first post with care, sharing what it felt like to live with HIV, the daily struggles, the misconceptions he faced, and the resilience he was finding within himself.

He poured his heart into each post, writing about topics that he wished others understood—how HIV had changed his self-image, how it felt to live under the shadow of stigma, and the strength he had found through his journey. The response was immediate and unexpected. His posts began receiving comments and messages from people who had experienced similar struggles, who thanked him for his words and for giving voice to their hidden fears.

Through the blog, Adrian found a way to educate others while healing himself. Each post became a small act of defiance, a way to reclaim his narrative from the grips of ignorance. He realized he was slowly dismantling the stigma by educating others, one reader at a time. Moreover, with each story he shared, he felt his strength growing, a quiet but powerful reminder that his voice mattered.

Family Dynamics

As Adrian continued to open up anonymously, he faced a more personal challenge: telling his family. His parents and siblings were supportive people, but they were also products of a generation and culture where HIV was often misunderstood. He feared their reaction, the possibility that they would see him differently, that they might feel ashamed or afraid for him. He had grown up in a household where specific topics were left unspoken, and HIV was one of those subjects that was rarely, if ever, mentioned.

After much deliberation, he decided it was time to tell them. He knew his family deserved to know, and he hoped their love would outweigh any fears or misconceptions they might have. With his heart pounding, he sat them down one evening and shared his truth. He spoke openly, explaining the medical facts, the journey he had been on, and his need for their understanding and support.

Their reactions were mixed, as he had anticipated. His mother looked at him with tears, overwhelmed with worry. His father sat silently, absorbing the information with a look of quiet sadness. His siblings seemed uncertain and hesitant, as if they were processing a world they had never known. However, amidst their varied reactions, there was love. They listened, they asked questions, and though they struggled to understand, they made an effort.

The experience was painful yet healing. Adrian realized their love was constant, while his family's understanding might not come quickly. This conversation began a new chapter in his relationship with them, based on honesty rather than secrecy. He saw that while their journey to understanding would be ongoing, he had planted the seeds of change. By sharing his story with them, he had begun to bridge the gap between fear and acceptance, opening the door to a relationship that could be deeper and more authentic than before.

Loyalty and Love

As Adrian's journey continued, he began to see who his real friends were. Some people in his life had faded away after learning about his diagnosis, unable or unwilling to look beyond the stigma. Others remained steadfast, their loyalty a beacon of comfort and hope. However, one stood out among the friends who stayed, offering support Adrian had never expected.

This friend, whom he had known for years, contacted him directly and compassionately. She listened without judgment, asked questions with genuine curiosity, and offered support without hesitation. Her presence in his life became a source of stability, a reminder that he was valued for his identity, not for any label or diagnosis.

Their friendship deepened as they shared more of themselves, and Adrian found that her acceptance helped him to accept himself further. Her loyalty reminded him that love could exist without conditions and that people saw him as he was, beyond any diagnosis. This unexpected allyship gave him the strength to continue his journey with renewed confidence. When given freely, he realized that loyalty and love could be powerful forces capable of lifting even the heaviest burdens.

Rising Above

With each new experience, Adrian's sense of self grew stronger. He began to understand that his value was not defined by HIV nor by the opinions of others. His diagnosis was part of his life, yes, but it was not the entirety of who he was. He had friends, family, and a community that stood by him, and he had a purpose that went beyond his struggles.

Adrian rose above the stigma that once held him captive through his blog, advocacy, and personal journey. He took pride in his strength, in the resilience that had carried him through moments of darkness. He saw he was more than a survivor—he could thrive, inspire others, and make a difference.

Rising above stigma became his mission, a way to reclaim the narrative around HIV, to show the world that people like him were not to be pitied or feared but to be respected. Adrian's journey had transformed him, revealing a strength he had not known he possessed. He had faced rejection, battled shame, and endured the loneliness of secrecy. However, in the end, he had found something far more powerful: the courage to live openly, proudly, and passionately commit to change.

As Chapter 4 closes, Adrian stands taller than before, no longer defined by society's views but by his resilience and determination. He has faced stigma, educated others, redefined his relationships, and risen above the world's judgments. With each step, he moves closer to a life defined not by his diagnosis but by the strength, love, and purpose he has found within himself.

Navigating Relationships

Dating with HIV

For Adrian, dating had always been an exciting part of life, a chance to connect, discover shared interests, and explore the possibility of love. But since his diagnosis, he found himself stepping carefully around the prospect of romance, cautious of the challenges he knew it would bring. As much as he longed for companionship, he feared the vulnerability that dating required and the courage it would take to tell someone that HIV was living with him.

His mind filled with questions that seemed to loop endlessly. Would anyone accept him fully, knowing his diagnosis? Would he have to face rejection repeatedly, his heart battered by the weight of truth he couldn't change? Despite these worries, Adrian decided he didn't want to give up on love. He still believed in the power of connection and companionship and was determined to find someone who could look beyond his diagnosis to see who he was.

The world of dating felt unfamiliar now. Adrian had to balance honesty with a sense of self-protection, carefully considering when and how to disclose his status. On early dates, he found himself holding back, hesitant to engage fully, constantly aware of the unseen weight he carried. He met kind people, others who were curious, and some who seemed to lose interest as soon as they sensed his guardedness. Each interaction was a reminder of the complexity of dating with HIV, a dance of caution and hope, of putting himself out there without revealing too much.

In time, Adrian began to understand that while rejection was a possibility, so was acceptance. His journey in dating became one of resilience, a lesson in perseverance and self-worth. He learned to view each experience as an opportunity to discover who he was and what he wanted, to find someone who would accept all of him—including the parts he once felt he needed to hide. As he continued navigating the dating world, he began to see that his diagnosis did not diminish his worth and that someone, somewhere, would see him for all he was.

Love and Boundaries

Eventually, Adrian met someone who made him feel seen in a way he hadn't experienced since his diagnosis. This person was gentle and attentive, asked questions thoughtfully, listened deeply, and respected Adrian's comfort level without judgment. Their connection grew gradually, a slow build that allowed Adrian to feel safe enough to open up, to let down his walls, one layer at a time.

As their relationship deepened, Adrian found himself facing new challenges—the delicate balance of love and boundaries. He wanted to share his life fully, to be vulnerable and transparent, yet he also needed to protect parts of himself and allow his healing journey to unfold at his own pace. The relationship tested his ability to set boundaries, be honest about his needs, and communicate his fears openly.

In this space, Adrian learned that love could coexist with boundaries and that he didn't have to give every part of himself to be worthy of affection. His partner respected his boundaries, never pressuring him to move faster than he was ready. This acceptance helped Adrian see that boundaries weren't barriers; they were a foundation for trust, a way to build a relationship rooted in mutual respect and understanding. Through this relationship, he discovered that love could be freeing and protective, a sanctuary where he could find strength without losing himself.

Trusting Again

Adrian's journey to trust was not easy. His diagnosis had left scars, and he had spent so much time protecting himself from rejection and pain that trust felt like an almost foreign concept. But with each conversation and moment of connection, he felt himself slowly opening up, allowing his partner to see parts of himself that he had hidden away.

Trusting again required a leap of faith, a willingness to believe that he could be loved despite his fears and insecurities. There were moments of doubt when he felt the urge to pull back, to shield himself from the risk of heartbreak. However, his partner's consistent patience and kindness helped him take those steps cautiously. Each moment of trust felt like a small victory, a reminder that he was capable of connection, of intimacy, even with the presence of HIV in his life.

In trusting his partner, Adrian found a freedom he hadn't known in years. He realized that by opening himself up, by sharing his fears and vulnerabilities, he wasn't becoming weaker—he was growing stronger. Trusting again allowed him to reclaim parts of himself he thought he'd lost, embrace the beauty of connection, and understand that true intimacy required courage and vulnerability.

The Weight of Disclosure

The question of when and how to disclose his status had always lingered in Adrian's mind, casting a shadow over his relationships and with this new partner, the moment had come to confront it fully, to face the weight of disclosure with honesty and integrity. He knew that this conversation would be pivotal, a defining moment that could shape the course of their relationship.

Adrian chose his words carefully, sharing his story, the journey he had been on, and how HIV had shaped his life. He explained his fears, the stigma he had faced, and the strength he had found along the way. His partner listened, absorbing every word, their face a mixture of empathy and understanding. When Adrian finished, there was a pause—a moment of silence that held a world of possibility.

To his relief, his partner reached out, taking his hand and offering words of acceptance that melted the tension Adrian had held onto for so long. They assured him that his diagnosis did not change the person he was and that they loved him entirely, without reservation. At that moment, Adrian felt a weight lift, a burden he hadn't even realized he'd been carrying. The fear of disclosure, of rejection, of being seen as less-than—those fears faded as he embraced the gift of acceptance that his partner had given him.

Breaking Down Barriers

In the following months, Adrian's relationship deepened, enriched by the honesty and trust they had built together. His partner's unwavering support renewed his faith in love, teaching him that he was worthy of acceptance and authentic, unconditional love. They navigated the challenges of his diagnosis together, each day reinforcing their commitment and respect for one another.

This relationship became a place where barriers melted away, where Adrian could be himself without the shadow of HIV looming over him. His partner's support helped him to feel whole, reminding him that love could break through even the most muscular walls. He no longer felt defined by his diagnosis; he felt liberated, empowered by the knowledge that he could be loved fully, without reservations or conditions.

With this love, Adrian felt a renewed sense of purpose, a drive to live authentically and openly, not just with his partner but with himself. The relationship became a mirror, reflecting to him the strength, resilience, and beauty he possessed. Adrian felt free to envision a future filled with love, hope, and possibility for the first time since his diagnosis.

As Chapter 5 concludes, Adrian has embarked on a journey of trust, vulnerability, and deep connection. He has faced the complexities of dating, the challenges of disclosure, and the need for boundaries, each experience helping him to grow and redefine his sense of self-worth. In this chapter, Adrian discovers that love can be a source of strength, a reminder that HIV does not define him but by the depth of his heart and the resilience of his spirit. He steps forward with a renewed faith in love, ready to embrace the life and relationships he once feared might be lost.

The Darkest Night

Relapse and Despair

Adrian had come so far in his journey—finding love, support, and a renewed sense of purpose. But with its unpredictable twists, life brought him to his knees once more. One morning, after noticing unusual symptoms, he went in for a check-up, hoping it would be nothing. But his doctor's expression told him otherwise. His viral load had unexpectedly spiked, and while his doctor assured him they could adjust his treatment, the news sent him spiraling into a fear he thought he had conquered.

This health scare shook him to his core. His mind raced, filling with questions and doubts he hadn't allowed himself to consider for a long time. The memories of his initial diagnosis resurfaced with a vengeance, the years of anxiety flooding back as though they had never left. For the first time in months, he felt the cold grip of despair closing in, whispering thoughts he had once worked so hard to silence.

The days that followed were some of the darkest Adrian had ever known. Each morning felt heavier, each moment suffused with impending doom. He questioned everything—the progress he'd made, the love he'd found, the advocacy he had embraced. It felt distant, like fragments of a life he was no longer sure he could hold onto. In the quiet hours of the night, he lay awake, his thoughts veering into dangerous places, wondering if he had the strength to keep going. The familiar fear of his body's betrayal left him helpless, and he began questioning whether he could continue fighting.

Haunted by Memories

As Adrian struggled to navigate this new wave of despair, memories from his past began to resurface with a vividness that left him shaken. Moments he thought he'd left behind now intertwined with his current fears, weaving a tapestry of pain that felt inescapable. He recalled the days after his initial diagnosis, the terror, the sense of isolation, the feeling of his life slipping through his fingers. But it wasn't only those memories that haunted him. Other, older wounds seemed to emerge as well—moments of rejection, childhood insecurities, and the deep-seated fears he had buried over the years.

These memories didn't come gently. They intruded on his thoughts like uninvited guests, each pulling him deeper into a place of sadness and regret. He relived the pain of friends who had turned away, family members who had struggled to understand, and moments when he doubted his own worth. He felt himself drowning in the weight of it all, the memories intertwining with his current despair, creating a spiral of thoughts that seemed impossible to escape.

With each flashback, Adrian felt he was losing pieces of himself. The progress he had made and the resilience he had built felt fragile, and he was quickly shattered by the force of his past traumas. He was no longer just a man facing HIV— he was a man facing the entirety of his life's pain, a weight that seemed too great to bear. The darkness around him grew thicker, and he wondered if he would ever find a way back to the light.

A Cry for Help

In a moment of intense vulnerability, Adrian reached a breaking point. He couldn't bear the weight of his thoughts any longer, and the isolation compounded his despair. Late one night, after hours of pacing his apartment, he picked up his phone and dialed a crisis hotline. He had never reached out in this way before, always priding himself on his independence and ability to handle his struggles on his own. But now, he knew he couldn't do it alone.

The voice on the other end was calm and warm, a lifeline in his desperation. He didn't know how to begin, stumbling over his words, unsure of how to express his pain. But the counselor's gentle prompts encouraged him to speak, to release the thoughts he had held inside for so long. He spoke of his fears, regrets, the memories that haunted him, and the despair that had taken root in his heart.

He let the total weight of his emotions come to the surface for the first time, unfiltered and raw. He spoke of his loneliness, of feeling like an outsider, of the dark thoughts that had plagued him for so long. The counselor listened without judgment, offering empathy and gentle reassurance. By the end of the call, Adrian felt a tiny flicker of relief—a sense that someone had seen his pain and understood. The conversation reminded him that he didn't have to carry this burden alone, that there were people who would stand by him, even in his darkest moments.

Holding on to Faith

In the days that followed, Adrian turned to his faith for comfort. Though he had always been quiet in his spirituality, he now found himself drawn to prayer and meditation, searching for a sense of peace he could hold onto amidst the chaos. Each morning, he would sit in silence, focusing on his breath, allowing himself to feel the presence of something greater than his pain.

Through prayer, he found small moments of comfort, a reminder of the inner strength that had carried him through his journey. His faith became a quiet companion, a source of solace that didn't demand anything from him but offered a space for healing. He recited prayers that his grandmother had taught him, words that now felt more meaningful than ever, carrying a promise of hope, connection, and a love that transcended his struggles.

In meditation, he found brief moments of stillness, pockets of peace that reminded him that he was more than his fears, more than his diagnosis. Though these moments were fleeting, they grounded him, offering a reprieve from the storm raging within. Faith became his anchor, a reminder that even in the darkest night, there was light to be found.

Reaching Out

As Adrian slowly regained his strength, he found himself drawn back to the connections he had formed along his journey. He began to reach out to others who had faced similar struggles, knowing that they, too, had likely experienced moments of despair. He reconnected with members of his support group, joining online meetings, sharing his experiences, and listening to the stories of others.

In these interactions, he found strength, a shared resilience that reminded him he was not alone in his pain. Each story he heard reflected a part of his journey, each person's resilience a testament to the human spirit's capacity to endure. Through these connections, Adrian began to see his pain in a new light as part of a larger narrative of survival, hope, and triumph over darkness.

The act of reaching out, of letting others into his experience, brought him a renewed sense of purpose. He realized that his story and struggles could offer hope to others on the same path. By connecting with those who understood his journey, he found healing in the simple act of being understood, of knowing that he didn't have to carry his burdens alone. Through this shared strength, Adrian found a way forward, a reminder that even in the darkest of nights, there was always the possibility of a new dawn.

As Chapter 6 concludes, Adrian has faced his darkest fears and emerged with renewed resilience. Though the journey has been painful, he has found strength in his faith, the connections he has built, and the act of reaching out for help. This chapter marks a turning point, a reminder that hope can be found even in the most challenging moments. Adrian's journey continues, guided by the lessons he has learned and the strength he has discovered within himself.

Newfound Purpose

A Community of Advocates

The turning point in Adrian's journey came when he discovered a community of people who shared his drive for change—a group of advocates who had dedicated their lives to breaking down the stigma surrounding HIV. This group wasn't just about support; it was about action. Their mission was to educate, empower, and shift the narratives that had long defined people with HIV. For the first time, Adrian found a place where his voice, experience, and passion could be channeled into something larger than himself.

He attended his first meeting with excitement and apprehension, unsure what to expect. The room was filled with people from all walks of life, each with a story and a palpable determination. There were those who had been fighting for years, seasoned advocates who had seen the movement's evolution, and newer members like him who had recently found their voice and purpose.

As he listened to their stories, Adrian felt a profound sense of belonging, a feeling he hadn't experienced before his diagnosis. These people understood his struggles, not just personally but socially and culturally. They had faced the same prejudices and battles and turned their pain into a source of strength. The room was filled with resilience and a shared purpose transcending individual struggles. In this group, Adrian found not only a community but a cause—a reason to keep fighting, a mission that made his journey feel meaningful.

Through his involvement in this advocacy group, Adrian began to see himself not only as someone living with HIV but as someone who could help others, someone who could make a difference. Each meeting and connection reinforced his commitment to this cause, and he felt his sense of purpose solidify, filling a void he hadn't even realized was there.

Using His Voice

With each passing week, Adrian became more involved and confident in sharing his story. He began attending events, speaking on panels, and participating in discussions that aimed to dismantle the myths and misconceptions surrounding HIV. Initially, he found public speaking intimidating. The thought of revealing his experience, of standing up in front of strangers to discuss his diagnosis, was daunting. Yet, each time he shared, his confidence grew, and his voice strengthened.

Adrian spoke about the challenges he had faced, the fear, the shame, and the resilience he had discovered along the way. He shared the loneliness, internal battles, moments of despair, and joy he had found in reclaiming his life. With every speech, he noticed his words' impact on those around him. People listened with empathy, nodding in understanding or surprise, some even shedding tears as he recounted his journey.

In these moments, Adrian realized that his story had the power to change minds, shift perspectives, and ignite compassion. His voice became a tool for healing—not only for himself but also for others fighting their battles. He saw that by speaking out, he could help others feel less alone, less defined by their diagnoses, and more empowered to live fully. Adrian's voice became a beacon, a symbol of resilience, and a reminder that while HIV might live with him, it did not control him.

Turning Pain into Power

One day, Adrian was invited to share his story publicly, beyond the safe spaces of support groups and advocacy meetings. This event was more significant, the audience was more diverse, and the stakes were higher. A familiar wave of anxiety washed over him as he stood backstage, waiting for his turn to speak. But beneath the nerves, there was something else—a sense of purpose that steadied him, reminding him why he was there.

When he stepped onto the stage, he felt the weight of his journey, the years of struggle, and the battles he had fought internally and externally. But instead of feeling heavy, his pain felt powerful, a source of strength that propelled him forward. He spoke honestly, sharing the moments that had shaped him, the lessons he had learned, and the hope he had found in his journey.

As he finished, the audience erupted in applause, but more importantly, he felt an internal shift—a transformation of his pain into purpose. At that moment, Adrian understood that his story was more than a personal journey; it was a tool for change, a way to educate, inspire, and advocate. His passion for this cause was ignited, and he knew he wanted to continue sharing and using his experiences as a catalyst for transformation. Adrian had turned his pain into power, and it fueled a newfound commitment to his mission of breaking down the barriers surrounding HIV.

An Unexpected Mentor

In his advocacy work, Adrian crossed paths with a seasoned advocate, a woman named Linda, who had been fighting stigma and advocating for HIV awareness for decades. Linda was wise, resilient, and unapologetically fierce in her pursuit of change. She had seen the movement evolve, had witnessed the losses and the victories, and had dedicated her life to ensuring that no one faced the struggles of HIV alone.

Linda took Adrian under her wing, offering him guidance, encouragement, and insights from her years of experience. She taught him strategies to stay mentally strong and cope with the inevitable challenges and criticisms of advocacy. She shared her stories of rejection, acceptance, and resilience to keep going even when it felt like the world wasn't listening.

Through Linda's mentorship, Adrian learned how to be a more effective advocate and care for himself along the way. She reminded him that while the work was essential, so was his well-being. She taught him the importance of balance, of finding moments of peace and joy amidst the struggle. Linda became a mentor, a friend, and a powerful reminder that he was part of a legacy of resilience, of people who had paved the way and were now passing the torch to him.

Building a Platform

Inspired by Linda's guidance and the impact he had seen from sharing his story, Adrian decided to build his own platform. He returned to writing, channeling his experiences, thoughts, and insights into a blog dedicated to spreading awareness and fostering understanding around HIV. This blog became his project, a space where he could educate, inspire, and connect with readers from all walks of life.

Adrian poured himself into each post, writing about topics that were both deeply personal and universally relevant—stigma, mental health, relationships, and the power of resilience. He shared his journey openly, offering advice, comfort, and solidarity to those who might be struggling in silence. His blog gained traction quickly, with readers drawn to his authenticity, courage, and determination to make a difference.

Through his blog, Adrian reached people beyond his immediate community, connecting with readers worldwide.

Each comment, message, and story shared by his readers reminded him of the importance of his mission. His platform became a space for healing and understanding, a place where people could learn, reflect, and find hope. By building this platform, Adrian solidified his role as an advocate, using his voice to create change, educate, and ensure that no one else would face their journey alone.

As Chapter 7 concludes, Adrian has fully embraced his purpose. He has found a community, discovered the power of his voice, and turned his pain into a catalyst for change. Through mentorship, advocacy, and his platform, he has built a life filled with meaning, resilience, and a commitment to making a difference. Adrian's journey is no longer just about surviving with HIV—it is about thriving, empowering others, and creating a world where everyone can live openly, proudly, and without fear.

Acceptance and Forgiveness

Self-Acceptance

Adrian had spent years wrestling with his diagnosis, the weight of it often pulling him between fear and resilience. Through his advocacy work, friendships, and growth journey, he began seeing himself in a new light. But now, he was starting to understand that true peace would require something more profound—a complete acceptance of his life as it was, without conditions or reservations.

In the quiet moments, Adrian would reflect on everything he had been through. His diagnosis was a part of him, yes, but it was not the entirety of who he was. He was still Adrian—the friend, the son, the advocate, the man with dreams and hopes, talents and quirks. HIV might live with him, but it was only one part of the more significant, complex, and beautiful story of his life. Slowly, he realized he didn't need to push away this part of himself or let it overshadow his identity. He could allow it space in his life, just as he allowed space for all his other experiences, joys, ambitions, and growth.

This journey to self-acceptance was a gradual process, marked by moments of clarity and doubt. There were days when he felt confident and grounded in his worth and purpose. And there were still days when he felt small, overwhelmed by the challenges that accompanied his diagnosis. But over time, he began to feel a deep, unshakable understanding that he was whole, exactly as he was. In all his strengths and struggles, accepting himself became the foundation upon which he could truly live.

Healing Old Wounds

With self-acceptance came the realization that Adrian had held onto certain emotions for too long. He knew he couldn't fully embrace his future until he had made peace with his past. Therapy had been a guiding light in this journey, where he could explore the memories, regrets, and pain lingering in his mind's corners. His therapist gently encouraged him to confront these old wounds to acknowledge the feelings he had tried to bury.

Much of his pain stemmed from guilt and anger—guilt over the ways he had once judged himself, anger at the people who had failed to understand, and frustration with a world that often saw his diagnosis before it saw him. Through therapy, Adrian could face these feelings directly, give them a name, and release them individually. The process was far from easy; each session felt like peeling back layers of himself, exposing raw emotions hidden for years.

One of the most complex parts of this journey was learning to forgive himself. He realized he had been his harshest critic and often blamed himself for things beyond his control. Accepting his imperfections and acknowledging his humanity allowed him to finally let go of the guilt he had carried. Adrian found profound relief in forgiving himself, a release from the weight of his expectations and judgments. This act of forgiveness marked a new chapter, a space where he could begin to heal fully and embrace his life with open arms.

Family Reconciliation

With his newfound acceptance, Adrian felt ready to bridge the gap between himself and his family. His relationship with them had always been marked by love, but his diagnosis had introduced a distance he couldn't ignore. Although he had told them the truth, he sensed that there were still unspoken fears and worries, questions left unasked, and emotions they hadn't yet processed.

One evening, he decided to sit down with his family and talk openly, inviting them to share their feelings and concerns. The conversation was raw and emotional, filled with tears, words of support, and moments of quiet understanding. His mother expressed her fears, her worry about his health, and her sadness at the thought of his struggles. His father, often the silent strength of the family, admitted that he hadn't known how to help and that he had struggled with feelings of helplessness.

Hearing their truths, Adrian realized that his family had carried their burdens and been on their journey of acceptance and understanding. The conversation brought them closer, allowing them to see one another fully without the walls that had once stood between them. Through this reconciliation, Adrian found a renewed sense of closeness, a reminder that love could transcend even the most profound challenges. His family's acceptance became a foundation upon which he could continue building a life of authenticity and connection.

Embracing Imperfection

As Adrian moved further along his journey of self-acceptance, he began to realize that he didn't need to be perfect to be worthy of love and happiness. For so long, he had held himself to an impossible standard, believing that he needed to be "strong" at all times and couldn't afford to falter or show weakness. But now, he understood that true strength was not about perfection—it was about resilience, about showing up each day, even when it was hard.

He began to embrace his imperfections, seeing them as part of what made him human, relatable, and honest. He allowed himself moments of vulnerability, recognizing that it was okay to ask for help, to feel afraid, and to make mistakes. This acceptance of his humanity gave him a newfound freedom and a sense of peace that allowed him to let go of the need for control.

Adrian also found that he could have more profound, meaningful connections through this process. By allowing himself to be imperfect, he permitted others to be honest around him, to show their vulnerabilities and fears. He saw that his worth was not tied to his ability to overcome every obstacle flawlessly but rather to his capacity to grow, learn, and live authentically.

A New Lease on Life

With forgiveness and acceptance guiding him, Adrian felt a lightness he hadn't known in years. The burden of shame, the weight of expectations, the guilt, and the anger had begun to fade, leaving space for hope, joy, and possibility. He felt he had been given a new lease on life, a chance to embrace his future without the shadows that had once held him back.

For the first time since his diagnosis, Adrian felt genuinely free—free to dream, to love, and to live without the constant reminder of what he could or couldn't do. He no longer felt the need to prove himself to others or himself. Instead, he focused on what brought him happiness, the relationships that enriched his life, and the purpose that continued to inspire him.

With this newfound peace, Adrian looked to the future with excitement rather than fear. He had reclaimed his life, not by erasing his struggles but by accepting them, learning from them, and allowing them to shape him into the person he had become. This chapter of forgiveness and acceptance marked the beginning of a new era, where Adrian could live fully and wholeheartedly, with a spirit unburdened by the past.

As Chapter 8 concludes, Adrian stands at the threshold of a new beginning. He has found acceptance in himself, healing in his past, and reconciliation with his family. His journey is no longer defined by struggle alone but by the profound peace he has found in forgiveness and the joy he feels in embracing life as it is. Adrian's journey continues, now guided by a deep sense of purpose, love, and self-acceptance that will carry him into the future.

Living Authentically

No More Secrets

As Adrian's journey continued, he found himself at a crossroads. For years, he had lived with the quiet burden of his diagnosis, carefully choosing whom to trust and navigating relationships with a sense of guardedness. But as he grew in self-acceptance and embraced his purpose, he felt the weight of secrecy begin to lift. He realized that the only way to live fully and freely was to shed the cloak of hiding, to allow himself to exist without the constant worry of others' judgments or assumptions. It was time to live without secrets.

Making this decision was no small step. The world could still be harsh and unforgiving, and he knew that transparency might invite questions, judgment, or even rejection. Yet, he also knew that he had reached a point where living authentically mattered more than the risk of misunderstanding. Each day, Adrian felt more aligned with his values and connected to his sense of self. He wanted to be known for who he was—entirely and without reservation.

Adrian began to share his story openly with friends, colleagues, and acquaintances, speaking about his journey not as a confession but as a declaration of his truth. Each conversation became a moment of liberation, a release from the constraints he had once imposed on himself. He felt lighter, as though the parts of him he had kept hidden were finally being integrated, finally allowed to breathe. Living authentically wasn't just about his diagnosis; it was about embracing every part of his life, knowing that he was enough just as he was.

The Power of Transparency

With each step into openness, Adrian found a profound freedom he had never known. Living without secrets allowed him to reclaim control over his narrative and define his story on his terms rather than letting fear dictate his choices. The act of transparency became a source of peace, affirming his strength and resilience. He no longer had to worry about hiding parts of himself or second-guessing how much to share. Instead, he confidently embraced his truth, unafraid of how others might respond.

Transparency offered Adrian a sense of clarity, a simplicity that he hadn't realized he was missing. By being honest about his journey, he no longer felt pressured to keep up a facade or compartmentalize his life. The boundaries between his personal and public selves began to dissolve, and he felt a newfound alignment with his core values. He was no longer living for others' approval; he was living for himself, for the truth of who he was.

This openness also invited others to share more openly with him. Friends and acquaintances responded compassionately, some even expressing admiration for his courage. And while not everyone understood or approved, Adrian could handle their reactions with a sense of peace. His confidence in his truth created a shield against judgment, allowing him to live fully, anchored in the power of his authenticity.

Strengthening Relationships

As Adrian embraced transparency, he saw a transformation in his relationships. The people closest to him responded with warmth and acceptance, and he found that his willingness to share had a ripple effect, encouraging others to open up about their struggles, fears, and dreams. Friends who had once known only parts of his story now saw him in his entirety, and his vulnerability created a space for deeper, more genuine connections.

Adrian felt a renewed closeness with his family, an intimacy that came from knowing there was nothing left to hide. His parents, siblings, and extended family members expressed gratitude for his openness, and their love felt more prosperous and complete. In sharing his whole self with them, he strengthened the bonds that held them together, weaving a new sense of trust and unity into their relationships.

This openness extended to new friendships as well. People who came into Adrian's life saw him as he was, without the walls he had once kept up. He found that he was no longer afraid of judgment or rejection; he was confident in his worth, and this confidence drew people to him. His relationships flourished, strengthened by his commitment to authenticity, and he discovered that by showing up fully, he was creating a life filled with genuine, supportive connections.

Advocacy Work

As Adrian's journey of authenticity deepened, so did his work in HIV advocacy. Now, he spoke not only as a community member but as someone fully open about his experiences, someone who had embraced his identity and found purpose in sharing his truth. His advocacy work gained momentum as he shared his story with larger audiences, raising awareness, fighting stigma, and promoting understanding.

He was invited to speak at conferences, community events, and schools, each opportunity allowing him to reach new people and challenge the misconceptions surrounding HIV. Adrian's story resonated with audiences, his words offering hope to those who felt isolated and educating those who had never understood the realities of living with HIV. His honesty broke down barriers, transforming strangers' fears into empathy and inspiring others to see beyond the diagnosis.

Adrian's advocacy extended to policy work as well. He joined efforts to improve healthcare access and fight discrimination, using his voice to push for systemic change. His platform continued to grow, and he became a respected figure in the community, known for his courage, empathy, and dedication. In this work, Adrian found a sense of purpose and a profound connection to others. Advocacy became more than just work; it became a mission, a commitment to create a world where everyone could live openly, authentically, and without fear.

Finding Joy

In living authentically, Adrian discovered a renewed sense of joy. Shedding the burden of secrecy and embracing his truth allowed him to reconnect with life's simple pleasures—the laughter of friends, the warmth of the sun on his face, the peace of a quiet morning. He found happiness in moments he had once overlooked, moments that reminded him of the beauty in simply being alive.

Adrian allowed himself to dream again, to imagine a future not limited by fear or shame. He pursued hobbies he loved, traveled to new places, and reconnected with his creativity. For the first time in years, he felt free to explore, try new things, and take risks without the nagging worry that had once held him back. Living fully had become his mantra, a promise to himself to embrace each day and experience with gratitude and presence.

This newfound joy didn't erase the challenges he faced, but it offered him resilience that made those challenges feel lighter. Adrian had learned to find peace within himself, to cherish the life he had, and to live each moment as a celebration of his journey. He understood now that his life was a gift in all its complexity and was determined to make the most of it.

As Chapter 9 concludes, Adrian stands as a man transformed. He has embraced authenticity, strengthened his relationships, and found joy in living fully, without secrets. His journey of self-acceptance, transparency, and purpose has brought him to a place of peace where he can look to the future with hope and excitement. Adrian's story is no longer about survival alone—it is about thriving, about building a life rich with meaning, connection, and a deep appreciation for every moment.

A Life Reclaimed

Embracing New Challenges

Adrian stood on the threshold of a new life shaped by the resilience, purpose, and authenticity he had discovered on his journey. For so long, he had lived in survival mode, focusing on simply getting through each day and each challenge. But now, he felt a shift within himself, a sense of readiness to embrace the future, not with fear but with hope and anticipation.

Living authentically had opened doors he hadn't even imagined. New opportunities emerged—more advocacy work, invitations to speak in places he'd once only dreamed of visiting, and collaborations with people who shared his passion for creating a more compassionate world. Each challenge he faced was no longer a burden but a chance to grow, a way to deepen his commitment to himself and his community. His past fears and insecurities had transformed into sources of strength, his doubts into stepping stones.

With every step forward, Adrian found himself more resilient and capable of facing whatever lay ahead. He saw each challenge as an opportunity to continue evolving, expand his impact, and live a life grounded in purpose. He welcomed it rather than fearing the unknown, knowing he had already overcome so much. The future was no longer a shadowed path; it was a wide-open landscape filled with possibilities, and he was ready to explore it with courage and joy.

Gratitude and Grace

In moments of reflection, Adrian felt a profound gratitude for his journey, including the struggles that once seemed insurmountable. He realized that every hardship, every moment of pain, had played a role in shaping him into the person he had become. His challenges had forced him to dig deeper, to find strength and compassion he hadn't known existed. His journey had shown him what it meant to truly live, embracing both the light and the dark gracefully.

Adrian felt gratitude not only for his growth but also for the people who had supported him along the way—his family, friends, mentors, and even strangers who had offered him kindness when he needed it most. Each of them had been a part of his healing, a part of the strength he now carried with him. Their love and support had helped him see his worth and believe in a future filled with hope and possibility.

This gratitude filled Adrian with a sense of peace, a quiet confidence that allowed him to face each day with openness and acceptance. He no longer felt defined by his diagnosis or the stigma he had once feared. Instead, he felt represented by the grace he had cultivated, the compassion he offered to others and his profound appreciation for the life he had reclaimed. Gratitude became his guiding force, a reminder that even in the darkest times, there was beauty to be found.

Empowering Others

Each day, Adrian felt an increasing desire to pay forward the support and wisdom he had received. He began mentoring others who were newly diagnosed, offering them the understanding, empathy, and encouragement that had once helped him find his way. These mentoring relationships became a cornerstone of his life, a way for him to transform his experiences into a source of hope for others.

He listened to their fears, validated their pain, and shared his journey openly, showing them that there was life beyond a diagnosis and that resilience and joy were possible. Adrian's mentorship wasn't about offering solutions; it was about being a compassionate presence who understood their struggles and could walk beside them as they found their paths forward.

Through this work, Adrian found a renewed sense of purpose. Each person he mentored reminded him of his journey, and each one inspired him to continue living with authenticity and courage. By empowering others, Adrian discovered that his story was not only his own—it was part of a larger narrative of resilience that connected him to countless others who were on their journeys of self-acceptance and healing. In helping others, he deepened his healing, and his life became a testament to the strength of giving back.

The Legacy of Resilience

As Adrian's story unfolded, he began to see his journey's impact on the people around him. His advocacy work, openness, and dedication to living authentically left a lasting mark on his community and beyond. People he had never met reached out, sharing how his story gave them hope and his resilience inspired them to rise above their struggles.

Adrian's legacy was one of courage, empathy, and unyielding resilience. He had faced the darkest parts of himself, confronted the stigma surrounding his diagnosis, and emerged as a powerful voice for change. His life was no longer defined by the challenges he had faced but by the strength he had cultivated, by the light he brought to others. Adrian had become more than an advocate; he had become a symbol of hope, a reminder that there was always a way forward, no matter the struggle.

His story became a beacon for others, an example of what it meant to reclaim one's life and live purposefully. His resilience's legacy extended beyond his own life, touching the lives of those who looked to him for inspiration. Adrian's journey was a reminder that it was possible to find strength, live with compassion, and make a difference in the world, even in the face of adversity.

A New Chapter Begins

With his journey of healing, acceptance, and advocacy behind him, Adrian stood at the beginning of a new chapter. He had come full circle, reclaiming his life and embracing a future he had shaped. The challenges he had faced had not disappeared, but they no longer held the same power over him. Instead, they had become part of his story, a foundation upon which he could build the next stage of his life.

Adrian's path was now filled with purpose, with dreams he was ready to pursue and a life he was excited to live. He knew there would be more obstacles and moments of doubt, but he also knew he had the strength to face them. His journey had taught him resilience, gratitude, and the power of living authentically. He was ready to step forward, guided by the lessons he had learned and the love he had found within himself.

As he embarked on this new chapter, Adrian felt a sense of freedom and peace. He had reclaimed his life, not as a survivor but as someone who had embraced his story, found his purpose, and transformed his pain into a source of strength. With a heart full of gratitude and an unbreakable spirit, Adrian set off on a path filled with hope, ready for whatever lay ahead.

As Chapter 10 concludes, Adrian's journey comes to a place of profound completion. He has embraced his challenges, found gratitude in his struggles, empowered others, and left a legacy of resilience and hope. With a new chapter awaiting him, Adrian steps forward with courage, ready to live a life of meaning, purpose, and joy. His story is one of transformation, a testament to the strength of the human spirit, and a reminder that life, in all its complexity, is a gift to be cherished and lived fully.

<div align="center">~~~~~~~~~~~~</div>

Invisible Strength: A Journey of Resilience with HIV is a fictional yet deeply authentic story that follows Adrian, a man whose life is transformed by an HIV diagnosis. Through ten poignant chapters, readers accompany Adrian from the initial shock and isolation of his diagnosis to his ultimate journey of self-acceptance, advocacy, and inner peace.

Adrian's story begins with raw vulnerability as he navigates the waves of fear, shame, and loneliness that follow his diagnosis. As he comes to terms with the realities of HIV, he faces prejudice and misunderstanding, both from society and from within himself. His journey is filled with challenges—from the daily weight of anxiety to moments of deep despair—but it is also marked by resilience, courage, and a steadfast search for hope.

As Adrian learns to live authentically, he finds strength in the support of friends, family, and a community of advocates who stand with him. Through advocacy and the power of his voice, he transforms his pain into a source of empowerment, becoming a voice for others who may feel silenced by stigma. Along the way, he discovers that living with HIV does not define him; instead, it becomes part of a larger story of healing, compassion, and purpose.

This book is an inspirational journey that speaks to anyone facing adversity or seeking the courage to live openly and truthfully. Adrian's story highlights the strength of self-acceptance, the healing power of connection, and the profound impact of living a life of purpose. *Invisible Strength* is a testament to the human spirit, a reminder that despite life's most significant challenges, there is always a path to resilience, joy, and self-discovery.

Author's Final Thoughts

Writing *Invisible Strength* has explored resilience, authenticity, and the power of human connection. This story, though fictional, is grounded in the experiences that so many individuals face—navigating a diagnosis, confronting stigma, and ultimately finding a way to reclaim their lives. Adrian's journey reflects that, while life's challenges may feel insurmountable, each of us possesses an inner strength that can guide us toward healing and purpose.

In sharing Adrian's story, I hope to offer a voice to those who feel unseen or silenced by the weight of judgment. Too often, the world fails to look beyond labels, allowing misunderstandings and prejudices to cloud our ability to see each other's humanity. But within each person, regardless of diagnosis or circumstance, lies a vibrant spirit, a story waiting to be told, and a life worthy of respect and compassion.

This journey reminds us that healing is rarely linear. It is a process that requires self-acceptance, forgiveness, and, above all, courage. I hope that Adrian's story reminds everyone facing their struggles that they are not alone. Whether through the support of friends, family, or a community of allies, there is always a path forward, always a way to transform our pain into something meaningful.

May *Invisible Strength* inspire you to live authentically, find purpose beyond fear, and embrace the power of connection. Our stories, experiences, and voices matter. They are, after all, the threads that bind us in our shared journey toward resilience and understanding. Thank you for being part of this journey with Adrian, and may his strength remind you of your own.

Love and Light,

Closing Prayer

Father God,

As we come to the end of this journey, we lift our hearts to You in gratitude and humility. Thank You, Father, for walking with us through each chapter of our lives and for Your unfailing presence in our times of struggle and joy. We recognize that every step of our journey, even the difficult and painful parts, has brought us closer to Your love and Your purpose for us.

Lord, we ask for Your continued strength and guidance as we move forward. Grant us the courage to face each day with grace, to accept ourselves fully, and to live with the confidence that we are loved and worthy in Your eyes. Help us to see ourselves not by the world's standards but by the beauty and resilience You have placed within us. May we remember that no diagnosis, label, or moment of weakness can separate us from Your love.

We lift those struggling, those who feel isolated or burdened by shame or fear. Surround them, Father, with Your comfort and peace. Place people in their lives who will offer support, understanding, and love, just as You call us to be there for one another. Strengthen them, Lord, and remind them that they are never alone and that You walk beside them every moment. Help them see their value through Your eyes and know they are loved unconditionally.

Father, teach us to live authentically and to embrace the story You have written for each of us. Let us be vessels of Your grace, spreading compassion, empathy, and light to those around us. May our journeys serve as testimonies of resilience and hope, and may we always be willing to lift others as You lift us.

We pray for the courage to be open, the wisdom to seek purpose in our struggles, and the strength to embrace every day as a gift. Fill us, Lord, with a spirit of gratitude and peace. Guide us as we share our stories, stand together in faith, and find joy in the journey ahead.

In all things, may our lives bring glory to You, Father. Thank You for Your endless love, faithfulness, and strength to rise above. We place our lives in Your hands, trusting in Your plan and resting in Your grace.

In Jesus' name, we pray, Amen. Amen. Amen.

Question & Answer

1. How does Adrian initially react to his HIV diagnosis, and what emotions does he experience?

Adrian's initial reaction to his HIV diagnosis is one of shock and disbelief. He is overwhelmed by a wave of emotions: fear, shame, confusion, and anger. He struggles to comprehend how his life changed drastically with just a few words. His mind spirals with questions about his future, relationships, and identity, feeling an immediate urge to isolate himself from those closest to him. Adrian's diagnosis introduces him to a new reality, and the rawness of his emotions reflects his uncertainty and the intense vulnerability of the early days of his journey.

---

2. In what ways does stigma affect Adrian's journey, and how does he confront it?

Stigma becomes a significant barrier in Adrian's journey, affecting his self-image and relationships. He internalizes societal judgments, initially feeling shame and fear of rejection. The turning point comes when he overhears discriminatory remarks and decides to confront them, which ignites his resolve to address stigma publicly. Adrian confronts misinformation and challenges negative perceptions by joining advocacy groups and sharing his story online. His advocacy educates others and empowers him as he reclaims his identity beyond society's labels, reinforcing his self-worth.

---

3. How does Adrian's support group contribute to his healing journey?

Adrian's support group becomes a cornerstone in his journey toward healing and self-acceptance. In this safe space, he meets others who understand his experiences firsthand, which allows him to feel seen and validated. Hearing stories of resilience from other members reminds Adrian that he isn't alone in his struggles, fostering a sense of belonging and solidarity. The group's support helps Adrian process his emotions, embrace his journey, and view his diagnosis as a more remarkable story rather than a defining limitation.

---

4. What role does Adrian's faith play in his journey, especially during his darkest moments?

Adrian's faith becomes a grounding force as he faces his lowest points. When he feels overwhelmed by despair and haunted by past traumas, he turns to prayer and meditation, seeking comfort in a spiritual connection. Faith gives Adrian inner strength and resilience, even when answers aren't immediate. Through prayer, he finds solace and a renewed sense of purpose, learning to trust in a more excellent plan and finding peace in moments of stillness. His faith reminds him that he is not alone in his journey, and it helps him move forward with courage.

---

5. How does Adrian's perspective on self-worth evolve throughout the book?

Initially, Adrian's self-worth is heavily impacted by his diagnosis, and he feels diminished by society's judgment and his fears. However, through therapy, support from friends and family, and his advocacy work, he begins to understand that his diagnosis doesn't define his value. By embracing his imperfections and vulnerabilities, he learns that self-worth comes from within. His journey teaches him that he is valuable not because of his struggles but because of his resilience, kindness, and authenticity. This newfound confidence allows Adrian to live fully and love himself without conditions.

---

6. How does Adrian's relationship with his family change after he shares his diagnosis with them?
When Adrian shares his diagnosis with his family, it initiates a journey of understanding and reconciliation. Though initially met with a mix of fear, sadness, and confusion, this transparency allows Adrian and his family to build a deeper bond based on honesty and acceptance. Their openness leads to previously avoided conversations, and his family gradually becomes a source of support rather than judgment. By allowing them to see his vulnerabilities, Adrian helps his family understand the realities of living with HIV, and this renewed closeness strengthens their love and connection.

---

7. What strategies does Adrian use to manage his mental health, especially during moments of anxiety and depression?
Adrian employs a variety of strategies to manage his mental health, including therapy, mindfulness practices, and reaching out for support. Therapy helps him process his feelings, providing tools to navigate complex emotions and identify thought patterns that contribute to his anxiety. He also practices meditation and prayer, finding brief moments of peace that help him reconnect with his inner strength. Additionally, Adrian turns to his support group and trusted friends for encouragement, knowing that shared understanding can alleviate feelings of isolation and despair.

8. How does mentorship influence Adrian's personal growth and advocacy work?

Mentorship is pivotal in Adrian's growth, especially when he meets Linda, a seasoned advocate. Linda's guidance teaches Adrian the importance of mental resilience, self-care, and balance within advocacy. Her experience helps him navigate his work's emotional demands while reminding him that vulnerability is a strength. Linda's mentorship instills in Adrian a deeper understanding of his role as an advocate and a mentor, shaping his approach to helping others with compassion, patience, and strength. This mentorship solidifies Adrian's commitment to his community and his well-being.

---

9. How does living authentically impact Adrian's relationships and sense of freedom?

Living authentically allows Adrian to build stronger, more meaningful relationships with his family, friends, and community. No longer weighed down by secrets, he can connect with others on a deeper level, inviting them to see his true self without fear of judgment. This openness also brings a sense of freedom and inner peace, as he no longer needs to hide parts of himself. By embracing transparency, Adrian creates a space for love, trust, and mutual respect in his relationships, and he discovers the power of authenticity as a source of resilience and joy.

---

10. How does Adrian's story leave a legacy of resilience, and what message does he hope to convey to others facing similar struggles?

Adrian's story leaves a legacy of resilience by showing that life with HIV can be filled with purpose, strength, and joy. Through his advocacy, he challenges stigma and educates others, using his voice to create a world where individuals with HIV are seen and valued. Adrian hopes to convey that resilience isn't about overcoming every struggle flawlessly; it's about facing challenges with courage, seeking support, and living authentically. His message is hope and empowerment, reminding others that they are not defined by their circumstances but by the strength and compassion they cultivate within themselves.

10 Powerful Scriptures

1. Isaiah 41:10

"So do not fear, for I am with you; do not be dismayed, for I am your God. I will strengthen, help, and uphold you with my righteous right hand."

This verse reassures us that God is always present, providing strength and support through every difficulty. When facing health challenges, it reminds us that God's sustaining hand is there to uphold us, no matter how hard the journey may seem.

---

2. Jeremiah 30:17

"'But I will restore you to health and heal your wounds,' declares the Lord."

Here, God's promise of healing and restoration reminds us of His power to mend physical and emotional wounds. This verse provides hope for recovery and repair, affirming that God cares deeply about our health and well-being.

---

3. Psalm 46:1-2

"God is our refuge and strength, an ever-present help in trouble. Therefore, we will not fear, though the earth give way and the mountains fall into the heart of the sea."

This scripture reminds us that God is our unshakable refuge, even in the face of overwhelming challenges. When health issues bring fear and uncertainty, we can lean on God as our constant source of strength and comfort.

---

4. 3 John 1:2

"Dear friend, I pray that you may enjoy good health and that all may go well with you, even as your soul is getting along well."

This verse includes a prayer for physical health and spiritual well-being. It reminds us that God desires Wholeness for us—not just in our bodies but also in our spirits as we draw closer to Him.

---

5. Philippians 4:13

"I can do all things through Christ who strengthens me."

This beloved verse reminds us of the strength and endurance we find in Christ. In times of physical or emotional weakness, God provides strength that transcends our limitations, empowering us to overcome obstacles with His help.

---

6. Psalm 34:18-19

"The Lord is close to the brokenhearted and saves those crushed in spirit. The righteous person may have many troubles, but the Lord delivers him from them all."

This passage reassures us that God is near to those who are suffering and promises deliverance. It reminds us that health struggles do not separate us from God's love—instead, He is closest to us in our moments of deepest need.

---

7. James 5:14-15

"Is anyone among you sick? Let them call the church elders to pray over them and anoint them with oil in the name of the Lord. And the prayer offered in faith will make the sick person well; the Lord will raise them."

This scripture emphasizes the power of prayer and the importance of community in times of illness. Through faith-filled prayer and support from others, God's healing power is present and active, offering hope and encouragement to those in need.

8. 2 Corinthians 12:9

"But he said, 'My grace is sufficient for you, for my power is made perfect in weakness.' Therefore, I will boast all the more gladly about my weaknesses so that Christ's power may rest on me."

This verse reminds us that our weaknesses allow God's power to shine through. When we are physically or emotionally weak, God's grace provides all we need, allowing His strength to be magnified in our lives.

9. Romans 8:28

"And we know that in all things God works for the good of those who love him, who have been called according to his purpose."

In times of health challenges, this verse assures us that God can bring good out of any situation. Even through struggles, God is at work, shaping our lives for His purpose and blessing us in ways we may not yet see.

10. Psalm 103:2-3

"Praise the Lord, my soul, and forget not all his benefits—who forgives all your sins and heals all your diseases."

This psalm powerfully reminds us of God's ability to heal and restore. As we give thanks and remember His blessings, we can find hope in knowing that God's healing power extends beyond our physical needs to encompass our entire being.

These scriptures provide comfort, hope, and strength to anyone facing health challenges. They remind us that God is aware of our struggles and is actively present in our lives, offering peace, healing, and the strength to overcome them.

Resources

1. AIDS Healthcare Foundation (AHF)

- **Contact Number**: +1 (323) 860-5200
- **Email Address**: info@aidshealth.org
- **Website**: www.aidshealth.org

2. The Trevor Project

- **Contact Number**: +1 (866) 488-7386 (24/7 Crisis Hotline)
- **Email Address**: info@thetrevorproject.org
- **Website**: www.thetrevorproject.org

3. Centers for Disease Control and Prevention (CDC) – HIV Resources

- **Contact Number**: +1 (800) 232-4636
- **Email Address**: cdcinfo@cdc.gov
- **Website**: www.cdc.gov/hiv

4. National Alliance on Mental Illness (NAMI)

- **Contact Number**: +1 (800) 950-NAMI (6264)
- **Email Address**: info@nami.org
- **Website**: www.nami.org

5. The Well Project (for women and girls living with HIV)

- **Contact Number**: Not available
- **Email Address**: info@thewellproject.org
- **Website**: www.thewellproject.org

6. POZ – Health, Life, and HIV Magazine

- **Contact Number**: +1 (212) 242-2163
- **Email Address**: editor-in-chief@poz.com
- **Website**: www.poz.com

7. Black AIDS Institute

- **Contact Number**: +1 (213) 353-3610
- **Email Address**: info@blackaids.org
- **Website**: www.blackaids.org

8. Planned Parenthood – HIV & STD Services

- **Contact Number**: +1 (800) 230-7526
- **Email Address**: info@plannedparenthood.org
- **Website**: www.plannedparenthood.org

9. Positive Women's Network – USA

- **Contact Number**: +1 (510) 681-1169
- **Email Address**: info@pwn-usa.org
- **Website**: www.pwn-usa.org

10. GLAAD – HIV/AIDS Awareness and Advocacy

- **Contact Number**: +1 (323) 933-2240
- **Email Address**: glaad@glaad.org
- **Website**: www.glaad.org

These organizations provide various services, from health and mental health support to HIV-specific resources and advocacy.

U.S. State's Health Department Contact Information

1. **Alabama Department of Public Health**
   - **Contact Number**: +1 (334) 206-5300
   - **Website**: www.alabamapublichealth.gov

2. **Alaska Department of Health and Social Services**
   - **Contact Number**: +1 (907) 269-7800
   - **Website**: www.dhss.alaska.gov

3. **Arizona Department of Health Services**
   - **Contact Number**: +1 (602) 542-1025
   - **Website**: www.azdhs.gov

4. **Arkansas Department of Health**
   - **Contact Number**: +1 (501) 661-2000
   - **Website**: www.healthy.arkansas.gov

5. **California Department of Public Health**
   - **Contact Number**: +1 (916) 558-1784
   - **Website**: www.cdph.ca.gov

6. **Colorado Department of Public Health & Environment**
   - **Contact Number**: +1 (303) 692-2000
   - **Website**: www.cdphe.state.co.us

7. **Connecticut Department of Public Health**
   - **Contact Number**: +1 (860) 509-8000

- o **Website**: www.portal.ct.gov/dph

8. **Delaware Division of Public Health**

    - o **Contact Number**: +1 (302) 744-4700

    - o **Website**: www.dhss.delaware.gov/dph

9. **Florida Department of Health**

    - o **Contact Number**: +1 (850) 245-4444

    - o **Website**: www.floridahealth.gov

10. **Georgia Department of Public Health**

    - o **Contact Number**: +1 (404) 657-2700

    - o **Website**: www.dph.georgia.gov

11. **Hawaii State Department of Health**

    - o **Contact Number**: +1 (808) 586-4400

    - o **Website**: www.health.hawaii.gov

12. **Idaho Department of Health and Welfare**

    - o **Contact Number**: +1 (208) 334-5500

    - o **Website**: www.healthandwelfare.idaho.gov

13. **Illinois Department of Public Health**

    - o **Contact Number**: +1 (217) 782-4977

    - o **Website**: www.dph.illinois.gov

14. **Indiana State Department of Health**

    - o **Contact Number**: +1 (317) 233-1325

    - o **Website**: www.in.gov/isdh

15. **Iowa Department of Public Health**

    - o **Contact Number**: +1 (515) 281-7689

- o **Website**: www.idph.iowa.gov

16. **Kansas Department of Health and Environment**
    - o **Contact Number**: +1 (785) 296-1500
    - o **Website**: www.kdheks.gov

17. **Kentucky Department for Public Health**
    - o **Contact Number**: +1 (502) 564-3970
    - o **Website**: www.chfs.ky.gov/agencies/dph

18. **Louisiana Department of Health**
    - o **Contact Number**: +1 (225) 342-9500
    - o **Website**: www.ldh.la.gov

19. **Maine Department of Health and Human Services**
    - o **Contact Number**: +1 (207) 287-3707
    - o **Website**: www.maine.gov/dhhs

20. **Maryland Department of Health**
    - o **Contact Number**: +1 (410) 767-6500
    - o **Website**: www.health.maryland.gov

21. **Massachusetts Department of Public Health**
    - o **Contact Number**: +1 (617) 624-6000
    - o **Website**: www.mass.gov/dph

22. **Michigan Department of Health and Human Services**
    - o **Contact Number**: +1 (517) 241-3740
    - o **Website**: www.michigan.gov/mdhhs

23. **Minnesota Department of Health**

   - **Contact Number:** +1 (651) 201-5000
   - **Website:** www.health.state.mn.us

24. **Mississippi State Department of Health**

   - **Contact Number:** +1 (601) 576-7400
   - **Website:** www.msdh.ms.gov

25. **Missouri Department of Health and Senior Services**

   - **Contact Number:** +1 (573) 751-6400
   - **Website:** www.health.mo.gov

26. **Montana Department of Public Health and Human Services**

   - **Contact Number:** +1 (406) 444-5622
   - **Website:** www.dphhs.mt.gov

27. **Nebraska Department of Health and Human Services**

   - **Contact Number:** +1 (402) 471-3121
   - **Website:** www.dhhs.ne.gov

28. **Nevada Division of Public and Behavioral Health**

   - **Contact Number:** +1 (775) 684-4200
   - **Website:** www.dpbh.nv.gov

29. **New Hampshire Department of Health and Human Services**

   - **Contact Number:** +1 (603) 271-9200

- o **Website**: www.dhhs.nh.gov

30. **New Jersey Department of Health**
    - o **Contact Number**: +1 (609) 292-7837
    - o **Website**: www.nj.gov/health

31. **New Mexico Department of Health**
    - o **Contact Number**: +1 (505) 827-2613
    - o **Website**: www.nmhealth.org

32. **New York State Department of Health**
    - o **Contact Number**: +1 (518) 474-2011
    - o **Website**: www.health.ny.gov

33. **North Carolina Department of Health and Human Services**
    - o **Contact Number**: +1 (919) 855-4800
    - o **Website**: www.ncdhhs.gov

34. **North Dakota Department of Health**
    - o **Contact Number**: +1 (701) 328-2372
    - o **Website**: www.health.nd.gov

35. **Ohio Department of Health**
    - o **Contact Number**: +1 (614) 466-3543
    - o **Website**: www.odh.ohio.gov

36. **Oklahoma State Department of Health**
    - o **Contact Number**: +1 (405) 271-5600
    - o **Website**: www.oklahoma.gov/health

37. **Oregon Health Authority**

- o **Contact Number**: +1 (503) 947-2340
- o **Website**: www.oregon.gov/oha

38. **Pennsylvania Department of Health**

- o **Contact Number**: +1 (717) 787-3350
- o **Website**: www.health.pa.gov

39. **Rhode Island Department of Health**

- o **Contact Number**: +1 (401) 222-5960
- o **Website**: www.health.ri.gov

40. **South Carolina Department of Health and Environmental Control**

- o **Contact Number**: +1 (803) 898-3432
- o **Website**: www.scdhec.gov

41. **South Dakota Department of Health**

- o **Contact Number**: +1 (605) 773-3361
- o **Website**: www.doh.sd.gov

42. **Tennessee Department of Health**

- o **Contact Number**: +1 (615) 741-3111
- o **Website**: www.tn.gov/health

43. **Texas Department of State Health Services**

- o **Contact Number**: +1 (512) 776-7111
- o **Website**: www.dshs.texas.gov

44. **Utah Department of Health**

- o **Contact Number**: +1 (801) 538-6003
- o **Website**: www.health.utah.gov

45. **Vermont Department of Health**

   o   **Contact Number**: +1 (802) 863-7200

   o   **Website**: www.healthvermont.gov

46. **Virginia Department of Health**

   o   **Contact Number**: +1 (804) 864-7000

   o   **Website**: www.vdh.virginia.gov

47. **Washington State Department of Health**

   o   **Contact Number**: +1 (360) 236-4501

   o   **Website**: www.doh.wa.gov

48. **West Virginia Department of Health and Human Resources**

   o   **Contact Number**: +1 (304) 558-0684

   o   **Website**: www.dhhr.wv.gov

49. **Wisconsin Department of Health Services**

   o   **Contact Number**: +1 (608) 266-1865

   o   **Website**: www.dhs.wisconsin.gov

50. **Wyoming Department of Health**

   o   **Contact Number**: +1 (307) 777-7656

   o   **Website**: www.health.wyo.gov

This list provides direct access to health departments for each U.S. state, offering valuable resources for individuals seeking health information, support, and services.